FIT DAD
FUN DAD

TERRANCE EVINS

FIT DAD
FUN DAD

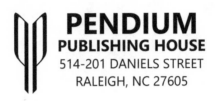

PENDIUM
PUBLISHING HOUSE
514-201 DANIELS STREET
RALEIGH, NC 27605

For information, please visit our Web site at
www.pendiumpublishing.com

PENDIUM Publishing and its logo
are registered trademarks.

Fit Dad Fun Dad
by Terrance Evins

ISBN: 978-1-944348-80-9

PUBLISHER'S NOTE

This book is printed on acid-free paper.

Chapter 1

My Style of Parenting

> "I am what time, circumstance, history, have made of me, certainly, but I am also, much more than that. So are we all." James Baldwin

I can't say I have a certain style. Maybe it's a mix of traditional and modern. I grew up in a non traditional way. Actually, it's more traditional now then the 70s-80s. I grew up with my father and step mom. So I was blessed to have 3 sets of families. Each, very different. Each taught me different lessons. Each loved me differently. There were days I didn't feel a part of any family and days I was a part of them all. But my glue was my dad.

I remember when it was just my Dad and I. He had taken a job in Elizabeth City as a dentist for the county. We lived on the second floor of a building that looked like it would fall apart. It was a studio apartment. The middle of the living room, we had a king size water bed! We slept in it together. But the inside wasn't the fun part. It was the view! We lived by the water. Actually it was Pasquotank River. We could see the Elizabeth City Bridge. So when boats would come in, I would stand there in awe as the bridge was slowly raised so the boats could come through. In front of our second story apartment was a huge field. We would throw frisbee for hours. I treasured those moments.

I learned then that it wasn't what was inside the home that made it a home, but it was my Dad that made memories with me so I could always enjoy the view.

What I learned from those times is the value of spending time with my son. I hope he treasures those moments. I hope that he sees more on the outside of our house then the inside. So my parenting style is really not a style I guess. It is more of sharing experience that he can recall and smile about when he becomes an adult.

3 Steps to Finding Your Parenting Style

1. Write out what you enjoyed about your childhood. What you didn't. What you learned. How you learned it. Figure out what type of father you want to be and if those ways will help paint the picture of yourself you want your kids to see.

2. Don't have a style at all! Adapt. Change. Learn. Your goal is to turn your child into a law abiding productive adult that can take care of themselves and give back to society. You want your kids to be respectful and not dependent on you. To feel love and know how to show love. How do you do that? It maybe different everyday!

3. Watch other parents and learn from them. Don't judge them but learn. You may see things or hear things you like. You may also see and hear things that you don't like. So, as the old saying goes, and learn.

Chapter 2

My Three Dads

I was blessed and lucky to have three Dads. Yes, I know that sounds crazy, but it's true! During times when not all kids have a positive male role model available, I had three! They were all role models to others as well!

My first Dad. Dr. Kenneth Evins (Doc)

He is not only my biological Dad, but he has also been an awesome role model. He has always been the person that I could trust and depend on.

I remember when I was very young. It was just me and my Dad. He had just graduated from dental school and took a job working in Elizabeth City, NC. Our first place was downtown Elizabeth city. We lived near the Elizabeth City Bridge and the Pasquotank Tank River. It was a one room studio apartment. The outside looked rundown and as you walked up the stairs to the studio, it was creepy with paint chipping off the sides. Our studio had a king size water bed in the middle of the room! It was great! Just us two! Outside thou, was the treat. There was an open field right across the street. It was off the river with views of the bridge. We could see ships and boats coming through. We saw seagulls flying over us all the time. We use to through frisbee and enjoy being outside together. Those memories helped shapes my view of my dad. He worked hard to provide for my sisters and I but what he provided that I remember the most are those moments. Us throwing frisbee and watching the ships. The sunsets over the river. He helped me view the value of time spent with the ones you love.

My Second Dad. ByungSeok Lee
(Master Lee/Sa Bum Nim)

I met Master Lee my freshman year in college. I had trained in martial arts before but when I witnessed a demo that he and Master Todd Harris did at East Carolina University, I was hooked! I was lucky that my training led me from classes with Master Harris at ECU, to classes at the main school with Grandmaster Lee. I was so excited, scared, nervous and intimidated! I remember that Master Lee didn't talk much. But he smiled and nodded often or frowned if something was wrong. He would carry a stick to assist in correcting your form. When he spoke, you had to listen carefully. But even if you didn't understand his words, you knew what he wanted through his body language. The language barrier wasn't ever a barrier! You understood every word, rather it was spoken in English or Korean! I remember after Saturday practices, we would gather in the lobby on the floor and eat together. Master Lee would tell us stories or just smile and stretch. I learned from him during those times how to be patient.

11

How to be gentle but firm. I learned that you had to listen with more then your ears when working with people. I also remember when Master Lee's daughter, Christina, was born. I watched how his whole life changed. I saw how much he loved his daughter and how much he and Mrs. Lee were a team. Mrs. Lee never worked at the school but she was more a part of it then anyone else. I saw how she supported him and even thou his days were long, she would be right there. Bringing Christina to the school to see him, and torment me! Bringing him lunch and snacks. From them, I learned the importance of family and building from the inside even when you are being pulled from the outside.

My third dad. Tommy Ellis. My Father-In-Law.

I met my wife my freshman year in college. I knew that she had a close relationship with her parents. Especially her father. I remember when I first had a chance to spend time with him and her mother. They came to Greenville and attended my 2nd Degree black belt test.

I was so nervous to perform in front of them. I wanted to impress them with my skills. Show them that Melissa had chose a person that could protect her! That test was one of my best ever! My forms, sparring were all on point. Then came my breaking. I was good doing board and brick breaking. My board breaking was a series of turning hook kicks fast, followed by a hurricane hook kick. My brick breaking was going to be a stack of 8-10 bricks to break. But Master Lee knew that would be too easy. So he changed it right there! It was going to be 6 bricks; 3 with each hand at The same time. Ok, no problem I thought. I remember Master Morgan setting up the bricks. He had put pencils in between as spacers. Master Lee looked at him, shook his head and said, NO SPACERS!! So a solid slab of three bricks!! Well, I didn't break it my first time. Or my second. On my third my hand slipped and I cut my wrist on the edge of the brick. Blood was everywhere! I still have the scar today by the way. But, I had broken one of them! The excitement that I only had two on one side, and three on the other to break, didn't last long. Master Lee instructed Master

Morgan to replace the broken brick with another! Now, I eventually broke the breaks. But I was also worried about what Melissa's parents thought. I remember her mom asking if I was ok. I remember her Dad saying good job but he didn't seem impressed! I knew I was going to have to do more to show him that I was going to be a good boyfriend(husband wasn't a thought at the time!) Eventually I think I did. Several months later, I visited Melissa at her house. I was sleeping on the coach. Her Dad and brother were headed to the barbershop. Out of obligation, I remember him asking me If I wanted to go get a haircut. I declined. I was bald headed! But I kicked myself when they went out the door because I knew I had missed an opportunity! But that didn't deter me. I kept coming around. Kept calling. I remember when I asked him if I could have his permission to marry his daughter. His first reply was it was about time! The second was that he only ask that I take care of her. For years I watched Mr. Ellis take care of Mrs. Ellis. They were always together. Traveling. Bowling. Eating. I saw them during holidays and regular days. There was never anything fake about their relationship or interaction. I saw them as the perfect family. In my mind then and still now they were the role model for parents supporting their kids. Melissa is a Daddy's girl and I am glad she is!! He taught her independence. He made her learn that she had to do things for herself. It taught me that I had to bring more to the table. That I had to learn how to support a strong women by being a strong man like her Dad. I am still working on it but the blue print he laid out is still visible for me to see.

The three lessons I learned from my Dads.

1. Spending time with the ones you love is priceless.

2. The way you show love is through actions not words.

3. Teach your kids to be independent and at the same time open for new possibilities.

Chapter 3

> "Impossibilities are merely things of which we have not learned, or which we do not wish to happen." Charles W. Chesnutt

Being A Dad

I always knew I would be a Dad. Never knew when. Or how. Actually, I do know how!! Maybe not how many. But I am a proud Dad of one. Now I have been around kids for ever! I have worked as a camp counselor, taught kids martial arts. I majored in Psychology and Child development while in college. I have always love working with kids and being around kids. So having one of my own, was a dream come true.

I remember when my wife, Melissa, told me she was pregnant. I had been out of the country for a couple weeks. When I returned, we were having a party for my birthday. We had a band, lots of alcohol and friends coming over. We were upstairs getting ready and she showed me the pregnancy test. I almost flipped! I asked if she was sure. She had already schedule to see her doctor but she was pretty sure. I was a mixture of excited, nervous and scared out of my mind! My thoughts were racing, not on what kind of father I would be but on could we afford a kid! I know! Wrong Thought. But that was running through my mind. Then it shifted from finances, to time. How would we schedule it all? Run a business? Spend time with a kid? Spend time with each other? I had seen and heard stories of how the wives spent so much time with the kids and both husband and wife forgot about spending time with each other. I didn't want that to be us. So, all of these thoughts are running through my head when guest arrives! What was funny about the whole evening was all of the red flags that some of our friends saw. The biggest, Melissa not drinking!! I went out and bought her a fake bottle of wine to have the appearance but that was quickly seen through. My friends Chryl and Kelli that had traveled from Raleigh knew something was up! The next morning at breakfast when Melissa didn't order a Mimosa, they definitely knew that something was up! My wife not having wine or mimosas surely meant she was either on medication or pregnant!! But those thoughts went away. My focus started being how I could be the best father I could be. My thoughts started going towards all of the positive father role models I had as well as the negative ones. I knew that I would be a disciplinarian but that I would also give my child (future Tyce), whatever he wanted! I knew I would be a mixture of softy and being hard. I also knew that I had to be his Father and not his friend. Knowing that I would have to sacrifice things to make sure he knew that I was there for him as a father. And that by being a father would be way more beneficial to him then being his friend. I am still working on being his father. There are always challenges but they change as he age. I find myself still with the same questions I had almost 10 years ago. Can I afford being a father finacially? The answer...NO! But we make it work because we can't afford not to! Do I have enough time to spend with him? The answer...No! But we make it work by scheduling the time. We plan vacations. We spend time together just he and I. I take him to school. Pick him up. I attend his school events and every once in awhile pop up for surprise visits. Owning a business gives me flexibility but it also limits my time that I have to them create to be a father. It's all about the creation! Being a father for me is all about creating memories daily that he can always look back on. I don't ever want to present myself to him as being perfect. I want him to see my flaws. But also see that he is my greatest gift. Now, did my wife and I stop spending time together and just focused on him? A little! But we figured out a balance that keeps us dating while being active parents in his life.

The Three things I have learned from Being a Dad.

1. You will always worry. It's what you do with the worry that matters.

2. Time is the most important thing to a child. You have to spend time and not just be there but be in the moment so they experience all of you.

3. Be creative. There is no written blue print on fatherhood. There are some awesome role models both positive and negative that will give you ideas on how to be a Father to your kid.

Chapter 4

"I am America. I am the part you won't recognize...get used to me...my name, not yours; my religion, not yours; my goals, my own..." Muhammad Ali

Fit Dad

Fitness has always been a part of my life. I haven't always been fit but I have had my moments! I have always been active. Football, baseball, basketball, track, martial arts. Even dancing! Have all been a part of my life. Yes, dancing! I was on the dance team in high school! Another story for another time!

I started training in martial arts when I was six years old. I trained with the same instructor who also became my football coach until I graduated high school. I tore ligaments in my ankle my senior year so my hopes of playing football in college was gone. But I still had martial arts. I remember when I was leaving for school, my Dad told me to make sure I find a place to train. He knew how martial arts kept me focus and balanced and how much I loved it. So I did. And I lucked out! I ended up at a demonstration that was being held for the ECU Tae Kwon Do Club. There, I saw Grandmaster Byung Lee and Master Todd Harris perform. I was hooked! I was in class that following Monday and never looked back. Not only was there a club to train, but there was also a competition team. And to top that off, it was covered through the school! So I trained. Daily. Including weekends. I traveled and competed and tournaments all over. Being a part of the ECU Tae Kwon Do Team become like being a part of my family. We trained until we bled. I use to limp back to my dorm after our sparring sessions. I iced some part of my body every night. And I loved every minute of it. I got use to the routine of working out daily. I got use to running miles daily. Running the steps of Brewster hall. I got used to conditioning on a canvas bag and taking licks from a bamboo sword. I got use to the bruises. The bloody knuckles. I got used to doing whatever it took to become a better martial artist. I also got use to not doing it alone. I got use to setting goals and achieving them. For instance, making weight was always crucial at a national competition. One year we drove about 14 hours to Louisiana to compete at Collegiate national. I was dead set on competing at a middle weight. So I had to be under 163lbs. The start of training was about 180. No real muscle. I put everything into dropping the weight. On that 14 hour drive, I ate nothing. Drank nothing. I remember getting in the long line to weigh in. Guys in plastic bags running and kicking to drop weight. I was dizzy, delirious and hungry! I remember stepping on the scale and honestly unsure if I had it. When the scale said 162.5, I was elated! I still have the badge that has my weight on it! The next day, we competed. And I won! So my goal of becoming a collegiate national champion became true.

That goal was one of many that I set for myself. I used my lessons of martial arts to help me achieve my goals in life, family and even more in my fitness goals.

I grew up watching my Dad play tennis on the weekend. Now he is an avid golfer. He was a fit Dad. I wanted to be the same. I am always challenging my self and reaching new levels of fitness. Why? Because I want my son to look at me and say that he wants to be a Fit Dad because of me. Kids do what they see us do. Not always what we tell them! Saying that I am a Fit Dad just motivates me to actually be one. And the cool thing is that we all can be. My goals of running half marathons, training in martial arts and doing body building shows are mine. We have to find our own and set goals to achieve them. I'm not done yet being a fit Dad. Mainly because my son isn't done with me being his father. He never will be!

What are the 3 ways that you can also be a Fit Dad.

1. Don't just set goals. Set outcomes. Visualize yourself achieving these outcomes and go after it!

2. Incorporate fitness into family activities. Work out together. Walk, run, jog, skip..something together! Let your kids see you go for a walk or to the gym so they know that fitness is important to you.

3. Be consistent. Life gets in the way. It always does. But don't use those road blocks as excuses to not be fit. Use them as motivation. Use them as fuel to work out more. Use them as motivation to be a role model for your kids. Doing a workout daily has become a part of me. Only because I was determined to be consistent. You have to do the same.

Chapter 5

"Any form of art is a form of power; it has impact, it can affect change – it can not only move us, it makes us move."
Ossie Davis

Balancing being Fit and Being a Dad

When I think about the word balance I tend to picture two people on opposite ends of a see saw. It's very hard to get that see saw balanced in the middle. Sometimes it's up and sometimes it's down. For me, that's how my life as a Fit Dad is. Now, calling myself fit may sound egotistical! It's actually more of what I strive to be. Daily. But, I fail at it. I fail at it a lot. The same to being a father. I fail at it. A lot. But unlike the instruction manuel that comes with the IKEA furniture, there is no step by step! All I have is an outcome of how I hope my kid will turn out. And daily, I have to strive for the goal. The same for being fit. I have a goal. Only on certain times of the year and certain times do I really hit that goal, but i do. Then I start over again reaching for you.

I remember when I decided to do my first body building show. Tyce was 3 years old. I was not in the best physical shape I wanted to be in. Now, I worked out all the time. I ran, did martial arts, I had just started CrossFit. But I wanted more. I wanted to look a certain way. Not just for myself but for him. For my wife. I wanted for her to think she had a hot husband with washboard abs. I wanted him to think he had a strong Dad that physically could tackle the world. Now I know that was all mental but for me it was motivation. So, I reached out to my trainer and decided to do a body building show. I was going to compete in Physique which was a new division. You wore board shorts instead of the bikinis. I wasn't ready for the bikinis! So, I jumped in. Full steam. Working out 2-3 times daily. Eating tilapia and asparagus 6 meals a day for 12 weeks. So, for 12 weeks, everything else took a back burner. There was no balance! No family trips. No weekend outing. No eating certain things at meal time. I was exhausted in the morning and exhausted at night. But, I had a goal in mind. So I competed in Physique in 2013. It was a great show. I placed 3rd in one event and 5th in another. I was proud of myself. So was my family. But I knew I had some make up to do! At the time, I knew this wouldn't be the last show. I had caught a bug. But I also knew that I needed to spend time with my wife and my son. I needed some weekend get always and family weekends. So, I took that time. Then I jumped back on the horse again. Fast forward six years later and I have competed in about 9 shows. My last two shows I finally wore those bikinis! I have also gone through hip replacement surgery. So that added to me not being able to balance. But, I did balance. For every show, there came time with my family. Time away. I have planed family time around show times and I have found a happy medium. My goal is only to compete one maybe two times a year. A compromise that is manageable for me and my family. And yes, my wife likes the washboard abs and Tyce thinks I can tackle the world. I'll take that balance!

3 Steps to Balancing Your life

1. Plan. Plan. Plan. Plan family times. Plan long vacation. Short vacation. Plan those things first then plan the other things around them.

2. Hold yourself Accountable. Make sure that you are fulfilling your end of the bargain. Communicate with your spouse and your kids to make sure that you guys are still on the same page.

3. Be Flexible. Always air on the side of family. Certain times in your kids life you can't get back. They are only at that age, that movement, that time once. Don't miss it!

Chapter 6

> "It is not light we need, but fire...not the gentle shower, but thunder. We need the storm, the whirlwind, and the earthquake." Frederick Douglass

Family Fun

So, how do we make fit, fun? We do that by making it a family affair. There is nothing like having your family behind your fitness goals. There is also nothing like having a family that have fitness goals of their own. Well, there is something that is better and that is having them together! Fitness is not a chore in our household. It's part of our everyday life. We live it. We eat it. We breathe it!

Even thou we have always been active, we haven't always been fit. For us, Fit is how you live your life. What you eat, do, breathe. Active is a part of that.

About 8 years ago I was in Australia. I was there for a martial arts training camp. I was there helping and training. It was my first time in Australia. Seeing all the site in Sydney, Melbourne, Balina, The Gold Coast, were all amazing! I met some awesome people that I still train with today. The camp was at a camp grounds by the beach. So we trained a lot on the beach. Meaning, we got wet and sandy and shirts came off. Again, I was always active. I trained martial arts, lifted weights. I thought I was rarely fit. We took lots of pictures. Training pics. One on one pics. I came back to the US feeling great about the experience. A few days later I was tagged in a picture by one of the campers. I looked at the picture and couldn't believe what I saw. I was FAT! At least in my eyes. I wasn't anywhere close to looking like I thought I looked or even what I wanted to look like. Everyone has always known me to be a bit stocky. I wasn't always. I competed in Tae

Kwon Do at 165lbs. Lean with no muscles! I graduated from college weighing about 190lbs. But now, I was fat! So, I called my friend who was a trainer and got my body fat done. I was 230lbs and 24% body fat! I had had shoulder surgery about a year before. Didn't push myself as much working out. I was teaching martial arts all the time but my body had gotten used to those workouts. So, I had gotten lazy and my past time was eating and drinking. My wife and I decided that we would both needed to make some lifestyle changes and both committed to becoming fit. I added in training sessions, then CrossFit. We went on a paleo diet. Then I went on a diet of nothing but tilapia and asparagus. I decided to do a show and went to the extreme. That extreme had me weighing in at 168lbs for first body building show. I was competing in physique. Wearing board shorts. I didn't have much muscle but I was proud of the 62lbs that I lost. Lots of it was water weight. But none the less it proved to me that I could do this. I could commit to a plan and stick to it. With the help of my wife and later my son, we became fit. To this day I still have those Fat pictures up that I see every morning. They are hanging on the mirror. It reminds me that that guy was me. But not who I am now. I have stayed committed. My goals change all the time. We tweak our diets. We indulge often. We are foodies that enjoy working off what we take in! We have embraced that we have to more consistent then not but getting off the tracks doesn't mean you can't get back on. My son is active in sports. He does martial arts. We do family workouts together. My wife does martial arts and Crossfit as well. She loves to cook and makes all our meals. The weekend we try new restaurants. But we don't stray from being fit. Today I still stay between 8-11% body fat. (I'm 9% as I write this!) I still do shows. My last show I weighed in at 173lbs and I was 4 1/2% body fat. Still working on improving that but not without the help of my family!

3 Steps to Make Fit, Fun

1. Plan active vacations. Hiking in the mountains. Throwing frisbee and football at the beach.

Swimming in the hotel pool. Walking the city streets exploring. Hit up a gym or the hotel gym early in the morning.

2. Enlist in sports. Have your kids play sports. Or join martial arts. You can practice with them during off time with the sport and even jump and train martial arts with them!

3. Indulge. It's ok to have that ice cream after a fun day running around the park. Enjoy that beer after your 3 mile run. Just done over indulge. Make sure that if you are going to have that ice cream or piece of cake then plan on how to work that off. For me, Sunday morning cycling class before church helps knock off Saturday night indulgence! But it's not every Saturday!

Chapter 7

"Success is the result of perfection, hard work, learning from failure, loyalty to those for whom you work and persistence." Colin Powell

How Do I Stay Fit

Getting fit. Staying fit. Both are challenges. It was just as hard to get fit as it is stay fit. But in order to do both, you have to set goals. Know what you want your outcome to be.

My first goal was to look good with my shirt off! That's it. I just wanted to go on vacation and hang out at the beach and the pool with my shirt off. I remember looking back at a picture from my honeymoon. We took a cruise. One of our stops was in Mexico. We hung out at the beach, drinking, soaking in the sun. It was beautiful. I even won a tequila shot contest! Ok, another story! We took a beautiful picture with another couple. I remember a couple years later looking at that picture. I was so chunky! I didn't look the way I wanted to look on the beach with my shirt off. I was thinking about how so many women go into a frenzy for there wedding wanting to look their best for their wedding. Melissa was perfect. And there I was a chunky mess! So, my first goal was to look good for her the next time we were on a beach in Mexico!

My next goal was to be a role model for my students. I was lucky that I had Grandmaster Lee as my mentor and role model. He defied age. He looked younger then he was. He always worked out and stretch. He was strong without having to lift a weight. And yes, he looked good in a bathing suit! I wanted my students to look at me the way I looked at them. I so wanted to be like Master Lee that I even bought a truck like his! Funny story. When I started training with Master Lee he had a black Toyota

Tacoma. He drove that truck everywhere and had it for ever. We hauled bricks and boards in the truck. Hopped on the back to go to demos. I said that if I ever open up a school, that I would have a black Tacoma as well. So a few years after opening, I found a 97 Toyota Tacoma. I loved that truck! I loved it even more because it made me feel like I was walking in Master Lees footsteps. Now all I had to do was look good in that bathing suit! I eventually did!

After we had Tyce, my fitness started to decline. I naturally wanted to spend time with him as well as be with Melissa. So working out daily took a back seat. I worked out but it was more like 3 times a week. I remember one day looking at him and thinking about so many parents I came across. They worked so hard to provide for their kids and doing things for themselves wasn't a priority. I understood. But I also understood that if I didn't get myself together that Tyce would see the things that I valued outside of him and that I wanted one of things to be fitness.

So, what did I do? I decided to challenge myself. I joined the Ultimate Black Belt which was a program created by Tom Callos to challenge martial artist to become better then they are both physically and spiritually. It was a test to have you change your way of thinking about martial arts and it's place I'm your life as well as your students and community. The test was a two year program that I had to have completed several requirements. Some of the requirements were journaling weekly online, doing 50,000 push ups and sits, sparring 1000 rounds, running 1000 miles, doing random acts of kindness, learning a new skills, becoming a white belt in a different style and more. The test was a challenge. We had to also travel to Alabama to help build houses for one of the poorest counties in Alabama. We went to Hawaii and trained with BJ Penn and worked on a farm. The final test was at Master Dave Kovar's school in Sacramento, CA. I remember on the trip to Hawaii a conversation with Master Tom Callos. He told me I was fat and I wasn't taken the challenge seriously! It pissed me off!! But deep down I knew he was right. I wasn't doing all I could. I was fatter then what I should have been. I took the words from him to heart. If he would have never been honest with me, I would have never decided to do all things I did after that. After that trip, I hired a running coach and decided I would run a half marathon. I got some of my students to join in. We all got hooked! I hated running but we made it fun by doing races in other cities. Over two years we ran about 12 half marathons. We ran in cities like Phoenix, San Antonio, Virginia Beach, Nashville, Miami and more. I went from running to CrossFit. From Crossfit to body building and I am still challenging myself. My son sees my medals and trophies and he wants them for himself now! He knows how important fitness is to our family. I know that he will follow in my footsteps in that aspect.

3 Steps to Staying Fit

1. Set Goals. Mark a date if in your calendar. Maybe that date is when you will fit into a pair of jeans or when you will run a 5K. Whatever it is. Make

that your first milestone and then plan how you will achieve your best fitness by then.

2. Get a mentor or trainer. Or both! Having someone to tell you the truth and help you along the way is key. You need someone to hold you accountable.

3. Tell everyone your date and your goal. Share with everyone that you are doing a 5K or you are going to your class reunion. Tell your family. Having the family behind you only motivates you more.

Chapter 8

> "We must combine the toughness of the serpent and the softness of the dove, a tough mind and a tender heart."
> Martin Luther King, Jr.

Where Do I Start?

I remember that being the question I asked myself. And I was so overwhelmed that I didn't know where to start. I remember coming back from the Tony Robins seminar. I was pumped about opening the school. I also knew I needed to loose some weight. So I went all in on eating the way that Tony mentioned. I started drinking a gallon a day of this green drink. I had cut out pork, chicken and beef. So, I became a pescatarian. I started back working out harder and trying to get myself back into shape. For several months, it had worked. Then one day

I went to a cook out. There was no fish on the grill. There was however some steak sizzling on the grill. It smelled wonderful! So, I had one! It was delicious! I decided then that I was adding steak back! But only a few times here and there. Now, after I had that steak, I got sick as I don't know what!!! You would have thought that feeling would have made me say that I was done, but it did the opposite. Made me say I need to eat more so I don't get so sick next time!

But, I started something. I started believing that I could achieved any task I set out for. I already knew that but this reaffirmed that. So, that diet wasn't for me, but adapting a healthier lifestyle was.

So, how do you start? Here are some steps.

1. Start with you. Being fit a lot of times means you have to be selfish. You have to take time for your self. You have to spend time exercising, eating right and meal prepping. Maybe at the beginning

the family isn't behind you because they follow by example. You have to set the example. You have to be consistent so they see that you are for real. It's not always a matter of support. It's a matter of them watching you to see if you are going to fail or succeed. They are rooting for you, but they may also be waiting! So be selfish. They will understand.

2. Incorporate your family. We talked about setting goals and sharing them. Now make sure your family is a part of it. If you are planning to do that 5K or Half marathon, invite them and make it a family affair. Your family needs to see that you set a goal, and you achieved it.

3. Have fun! Remember that the time you spend with your family, you can give back. Your kids are only at those ages for a certain amount of time. They go from sitting on your lap to barely wanting to hug you! So, have fun incorporating

a fit life. It's something you can do together always! Kids don't grow out of fitness. They may adapt a different way or a new sport. But fitness can always be what you share. Those moments create memories. So have fun!

Fit Dad Fun Dad

The workouts….
Plus some stories!

Obstacles don't have to stop you. If you run into a wall, don't turn around and give up. Figure out how to climb it, go through it, or work around it. – Michael Jordan

I enjoy working out. Actually, I love it! It comes third in my life. Family, business...working out! Working out helps me clear my mind. Helps me focus. I get the mental clarity with the physical benefits. I am not sure what working out does for you. Not sure where you are in your fitness goals. But I am sure that if you are reading these words, that you are looking for something. Maybe you are looking for workouts to follow. Maybe you are looking for workouts to give you inspiration so you can do your own workouts. Maybe you are just beginning. Maybe you are seasoned. None the less, we are all in this together. I am in this for you. You are in this for me. And together along with our family, friends and community, we can change this world, one push up, one burpee, one squat at a time! So enjoy the workouts. Use them. Create your own. Share them. Have fun with them. Alright, lets sweat!

Workout 1

Static Hold

2 Rounds

Round 1

Wall sit for 1 minute. Rest 15 Seconds. Max out air squats
for 1 minute

High plank for 1 minute. Rest 15 Seconds. Max out push
ups for 1 minute

Superman hold for 1 minute. Rest 15 seconds. Max Lat
pulls from super man.

Rest 1 minute

Round 2

Same as Round 1

Workout 2

Stair Workout

2 Rounds. 1 minute Each.

Step ups

Step up squats

Step up push ups

Dips

Sit ups

Repeat

Workout 3

Burpee/Push Up Ladder

30 Burpees-10 push ups

25 Burpees- 15 push ups

20 burpees- 20 push ups

15 Burpees- 25 push ups

10 Burpees- 30 Push ups

I hated every minute of training, but I said, 'Don't quit. Suffer now and live the rest of your life a champion'.

– Muhammad Ali

Book bag workouts. I know. A book bag. Quick story. My son Tyce was walking to the door with his book bag.

I called myself helping him. I grabbed his book bag. It was heavy! I asked, what is in there? He is only in the 5th grade. Cant imagine how heavy it will be in high school. Come to think about it, it was about as heavy as my wife purse!

Workout 4

Book Bag Workout 1

> Bookbag on your back. Have as many books for weight that you can handle.
>
> 15 Minute AMRAP (As Many Rounds As Possible)
>
> 10 Push Ups
>
> 20 Mountain Climbers
>
> 30 Air Squats

Workout 5

Book Bag Workout 2

> Holding the Book Bag
>
> 4 Rounds
>
> 15 Goblet Squat Squat hugging book bag
>
> 15 Swings to overhead

15 lunges (holding book bag over head)

15 Mountain Climbers

15 Leg lifts

Workout 6

500 Reps Total. Have to do at least 10 reps of each. After

that, then however you want want.

Push ups

Sit ups

Burpees

Air Squats

Lunges

Never let your head hang down. Never give up and sit down and grieve. Find another way. – Satchel Paige

I love pizza. I love burgers. Those are two of my favorite cheat meals. My favorite pizza place is... well actually it is a tie between three places. Alino's, Inizio, and Pure pizza. For burgers my favorite spots are Barcelona and

Alexander Michaels. I know I think about food a lot. I enjoy my cheats. But I work for them. We meal prep two to three times per week. We make sure that we eat a healthy and balance meals most days. So, when those cheat days come around, we enjoy! But for now, lets Sweat!

Here is one of my favorite body weight Crossfit Workouts.

Workout 7

Cindy

    20 minutes of:

    5 Pull Ups

    10 Push ups

    15 Air Squats

Workout 8

21-15-9

In and Out Squats

    Plyo Push ups

    Plank Toe Touches

    Do each exercise for 21 reps. Then 15 reps. Then 9.

Workout 9

5 Rounds

   10 Burpee

   20 Jack Squats

   30 Sit ups

There may be people that have more talent than you, but there's no excuse for anyone to work harder than you do. – Derek Jeter

I loved playing sports growing up. I played baseball, football, basketball and ran track. I was never the most gifted athlete on the field or court. But I was always one of the hardest working ones. If I couldn't beat you with speed, I would wear you down with stamina and heart. I had the best coaches growing up. My favorite coach however was Coach Capps. Everyone loved Coach Capps! Whether you played football, was in the weight room or not, you loved Coach Capps! Coach Capps taught us all about having heart. Playing with passion. Working hard. Not giving up. He didn't just talk about thou, he would show you if he had to as well! I remember one time he was getting on the offensive line about blocking. He kept telling us to get our nose into their chest, stay low and our hand up under the pads and drive them back. He got so mad, he threw off his hat. Lined up on the line. Blew the whistle and when the defensive guy, now remember, we all had on full pads. He didn't! He hit the defensive guy so hard, driving his nose into his chest that he busted his nose. Blood running down and he didn't even flinch. Kept fussing and grabbed his hat and told us to do it again! I have always aspired to have that type of passion in everything I do. That passion in every person that I teach and I coach. I learned that from Coach Capps.

Workout 10

5 Rounds of:

    10 Hand Release Push ups

    20 Side Lunges

    30 Double Cruches

Workout 11

15 minute AMRAP (As Many Rounds/Reps As Possible)

    20 Air squats

    10 Push Ups

    10 Chair Dips

Workout 12

3 Rounds

    50 Double Unders (100 Singles)

    50 Double Crunches

> **"Life is not a spectator sport. If you're going to spend your whole life in the grandstand just watching what goes on, in my opinion you're wasting your life."**
> **– Jackie Robinson**

I love Disney. Since Tyce turned 4, we have done something Disney related every year. Disney cruise, parks, ect. I even celebrated my 40th birthday party there. There is something real for me when it comes to the magic of Disney. Yes, its expensive. Yes, its a lot of walking. Yes, its expensive. Ok, I said that already! But for me, for my family, its the memories. Not saying that you have to go to Disney to make memories. Family time is important. So creating that Disney mindset, no matter where you are at, is key. I know that I only have a few more years with Tyce at that stage. I hope these memories and these times will have him wanting to spend time with us no matter his age. No matter if it is Disney or time at home. But I do love Disney!

Workout Time!

Workout 13

4 Rounds of:

>10 Quad Push Ups
>
>20 Plank toe touches
>
>30 Running Knee Lunge
>
>40 In and Out Air squats

Workout 14

3 Rounds

>20 Lunges
>
>20 Push ups/Alternating Knee up (Spiderman push ups)
>
>20 Plank Toe Touches

Workout 15

50-40-30-20-10

>Alternating Sit Ups and Air Squats
>
>50 sit ups, 50 air squats, 40 sit ups, 40 air squats etc..

> **"I think the good and the great are only separated by the willingness to sacrifice." – Kareem Abdul-Jabbar**

I have to workout in the morning. It is something about waking up, getting it in that really sets the tone for my day. When I don't get in that morning sweat, I feel it. I think everyone around me feels it to! Plus, no matter how busy my day turns out, at least I got in a workout!

Workout 16

Farmers Carry Workout using two Cinder Blocks:

Farmers Carry(1oo meters)

50 toe taps on the cinder block

Farmers Carry (100 meters)

50 High plank hand step up onto the cinder blocks

Farmers Carry (100 meters)

50 High Planks Knee ups (hop both knees in and back out into plank)

Farmers Carry (100 meters)

50 Push ups with feet on the cinder blocks

Workout 17

5 Rounds

   1 Min Plank Hold

   400 meter run (or run for 2 minutes in place or distance)

Workout 18

1 Mile Run

   After Run, Max Air squats into revers lunge

> **"It doesn't matter what your background is and where you come from, if you have dreams and goals, that's all that matters." – Serena Williams**

I love martial arts. I started when I was 6 years old. Almost 40 years later, it is still a huge part of my life. Talk about sticking to something! When I was 6, my goal wasn't to get a black black. It was just to have fun! My goal was to be like Bruce Leroy! If you don't know who he is, stop right now, and go watch Barry Gordy's Last Dragon! Anyway.. I am still on my quest for the final level and hoping that one day I will get the glow! Again, watch Last Dragon and you will get that last sentence! Ok, lets workout!

Workout 19

4 Rounds

    10 Quad Push ups

    20 Plank Toe Touches

    30 running knee lunges

    40 In and out squats

Workout 20

15 minute AMRAP

    15 Air Squats- 5 Second hold at 90 degrees for 5 seconds.

    15 Push ups- 5 Second hold at half push up for 5 seconds.

    15 Sit ups- 5 Second hold at half rep of sit up for 5 seconds.

Workout 21

3 Rounds

    15 Burpees

    20 Air Squats

    25 Jumping Jacks

    30 Sit ups

> **"Obstacles don't have to stop you. If you run into a wall, don't turn around and give up. Figure out how to climb it, go through it, or work around it."**
> **– Michael Jordan**

I remember when I did my first obstacle course race. I have only down a few. I have down the Warrior Dash a couple times and the Spartan Race. I was so ready to jump in do races everywhere that I even signed up for the Warrior Dash in Australia! My hip stopped me from pursuing that, but I learned so much about myself doing those races. Everything about those obstacles was a metaphor for our life. Hey, sometimes you have to tread through mud, or water up to your neck to get to the other side. Sometimes you have climb one wall. To get to another wall that you have to get over. To even another wall! Some days you are crawling under bob wire and others you are jumping over fire. But no matter the obstacle, or how muddy you get, there is always water to wash off the mud, even if you have to bring your own, and a cold beer waiting for you to celebrate with family and friends!

Workout 22

Chipper

    100 High Knees in place

    80 Double Under jump rope/or 160 single under

    60 Mountain climbers

    40 Plyo Lunges

    20 Bicycle crunches

    10 Triangle Push Ups

Workout 23

    300 Single Jump Rope

    200 Kettle Bell Swings

100 Plank Shoulder Touches

60 Second Wall Sit

Workout 24

15 Minute AMRAP (As Many Reps/Rounds As Possible)

10 Push ups

10 Twisting Mountain Climbers

10 Alternating Lunge to knee up and jump

10 Air Squats

> **"We all have dreams. But in order to make dreams come into reality, it takes an awful lot of determination, dedication, discipline, and effort." – Jesse Owens**

About 18 years ago I went to a Tony Robbins convention in Miami, Florida. It was called "Unleash The Power Within". At the time I had been laid off from my job. I was interviewing for positions in Pharmaceutical Sales. I was newly married. Had just bought a house. So, finding a job, making good income was top priority. Then something happened. I walked across fire, caught an internal flame and decided to open up my own martial arts school. Crazy! I visualized my first group of students. I saw their faces. I saw them in uniform. I could hear their yells and see the sweat dripping on my mats. A year later, those first group of students entered. They were just as I envisioned them! My dream came true. But the dream takes work. It takes determination, dedication, discipline and continued effort. I would trade it for anything!

Workout 25

100 Jack Squats

80 Lunges

60 Plank Jacks

40 Push ups

20 V sit ups

10 Burpees

Workout 26

3 Rounds

    400 meter run (run for 90 seconds)

    50 Air squats

30 push ups

15 Super man lat pulls

Workout 27

Descending Ladder of Burpees and Sit ups

10-9-8-7-6-5-4-3-2-1

"**Be the hardest working person you can be. That's how you separate yourself from the competition.**"
– Stephen Curry

I love working out. I love spending time with family. I love being a father. I love being a husband. I love being a son. I love being a brother. I love being a business owner. I love being a mentor. I love the things that I am strong at. I love the things that give me challenges. I love growth. I love failure. I love success after failure. I love all the different parts of me that make me, me. I draw from each of these things to fuel my workouts. To fuel my ambitions. Every day we all have to deal with some elements of ourselves that we need to celebrate.

Elements that we need fix and make better. That is what staying active does for me. It is window to how my life really is. Some days are better then others, but I still push through. You can still push through. You have before. You can now! Any way, that is my two cents! Now, lets sweat!

Workout 28

1 minute each exercise. No rest between exercise. 1 minute rest between rounds.

Round 1

    Air Squats

    Push Ups

    Mountain Climbers

    Sit ups

    Rest 1 Minute

Round 2

    In and Out Squats

    Plyo Push ups

    Plank Jacks/In and Out

Leg Flutters

Rest 1 minute

Round 3

Air Squats into Lunges

Quad Push ups

Burpees

V Sit Ups

Workout 29

4 Rounds

25 Jumping Squats

Workout 30

5 Rounds of 50 Air Squats. Rest in between each round the time it took you to complete the 50.

There you go! 30 workouts to get you going! Do them in any order you like. For reference of the workout and more workout inspiration, join our Facebook group, Fit Dad Fun Dad and follow me on IG!